The Ultimate Challenge
Is To Live Healthy

Publisher: Createspace.com
(An Amazon.com Company)
ISBN: 143824648X
ISBN-13: 9781438246482

~
Take it one step at a time
Let's Go!
~

Use Your Common Sense to Loss Weight

- ❖ Achieving and maintaining a healthy weight doesn't have to be a struggle. And it certainly doesn't mean denying your body the nutrients it needs to keep you feeling strong and healthy. Even small changes of habit can make a real and lasting impact over time.

- ❖ Set a reasonable weight goal.

- ❖ Losing weight at a slow steady pace can help ensure that the weight loss is permanent. Flip flopping back and forth is unhealthy for you, and causes you to fall off the wagon more often.

- ❖ If you loss the weight too fast it could come back, and That's Very Unhealthy!

- ❖ Think healthier, and the health benefits could be a lower blood pressure, blood cholesterol, and reduced risk of diabetes and heart disease

- ❖ A healthy and reasonable calorie goal for weight loss is generally 10 times your "goal" weight (for example, 10 X 150 pounds = 1500 calories). Add at least 10% if you exercise regularly

- ❖ Keep a daily written record of what you eat and drink – you may be surprised by what you're actually consuming.

- ❖ Recording fat grams and/or calories if you prefer, but a simple list should be enough to do the trick

- ❖ Enjoy some moderate physical activity every day – a 30 minute walk is fine.

- ❖ Exercise is the key to long-term weight control

❖ Substitute Smart Balance Light Buttery Spread on bread or toast and for light cooking; substitute fat-free or reduced-fat salad dressings for regular salad dressings. Substitute fruit for desserts

❖ Try to avoid bread with meals that include potatoes, rice, or pasta – Trust me you won't miss it.

❖ Choose water or a no-calorie beverage with meals.

❖ Watch your use of sweetened beverages and sodas, and watch the alcoholic beverages intake.

Your First Step:

Living Healthy!

It's a Simple Thing!

It seems hard to lose weight, when you don't know what you need, or where to start.

You can't think what children must go through!

With this Journal:

You & your family can take off a few extra pounds.

The steps are Simple, and the recipes are delicious.

From a simple and delicious trail mix, to a yummy shepherd's pie.

You & the family will live healthier and you will lose a few extra pounds.

Where to 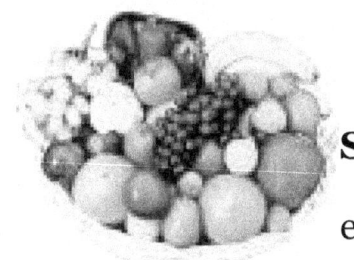 Start:

For me it was easy!!!!

I had a conversation with my family and I told them:
I'm 44 years young, and I want to stay that way.
But to do so I must change some things in my life.
  1. being the way I cook & eat
  2. I must add some exercise to my schedule
Now, you can join me or eat out.
"Thank Heavens They Joined Me"

So, I emptied out the refrigerator of all unhealthy foods;
I cleaned out the cabinets and donated everything that was
unhealthy or bad for me.
Then I went shopping & brought a Countertop grill, a Smoothie
Maker, and a good chopping board.

- I filled the refrigerator with fresh fruit and vegetables,
- Juices instead of soda and (but not too much juice either,
  sugar levels are higher can soda sugar levels, that's why
  you need to drink water instead)
- Bottled water instead of kool-aid
- Drinking green tea will help promote weight loss (more on
  green tea later)
- Skim milk or 2% milk
- Low fat cheeses
- ICBINB-I can't believe it's not butter instead of butter or
  smart balance margarine.
- Olive Oil instead of vegetable oils (Use Great tasting-
  Smart Balance Oil made with Canola , Soy and Olive oils)
- Ms Dash comes in several varieties, use it instead of salt
- Use low fat yogurt instead of milk in your recipes.
- Most importantly, you have to learn to read your labels,
  know what you're eating.
  When reading your labels always look for:

Lower fats,   Lower sodium   Lower Carbohydrates
Low Sugar   Vitamins & minerals

Read your food labels before you buy

Becoming smart shoppers by reading and comparing food labels to find out more about the foods you eat.

The "Nutrition Facts" panel found on most food labels can help you determine which foods are good sources of fiber, calcium, iron, and vitamin C, and which foods are lower in fat, calories, sodium and sugar.

But before you pack your cart with cans and packages touting various nutritional benefits and health claims, understand this: The U.S. Food and Drug Administration has strict guidelines on how certain terms on food labels can be used.

Here's the low-down on what those terms really mean:

- **Low calorie** – Less than 40 calories per serving
- **Low cholesterol** – Less than 20 mg of cholesterol and 2 gm or less of saturated fat per serving
- **Reduced** – 25% less of the specified nutrient or calories than the usual product
- **Good source of** – Provides at least 10% of the Daily Value of a particular vitamin or nutrient per serving (see below for Daily Value info)
- **Calorie free** – Less than 5 calories per serving
- **Fat free / sugar free** – Less than 1/2 gram of fat or sugar per serving
- **Low sodium** – Less than 140 mg of sodium per serving
- **High in** – Provides 20% or more of the Daily Value of a specified nutrient per serving
- **High fiber** – 5 or more grams of fiber per serving

The FDA also sets standards for health-related claims on food labels to help consumers identify foods that are rich in nutrients and may help to reduce their risk for certain diseases.

For example, health claims may highlight the link between calcium and osteoporosis, fiber and heart disease, and sodium and hypertension.

Here's how to read "Nutrition Facts" labels:

Serving Size
A serving size is the amount of food for one serving, or the number of servings in the package. Remember to check your portion size to the serving size listed on the label. If the label serving size is one cup and you eat two cups, you're getting twice the calories, fat and other nutrients listed on the label.

Total Calories and Fat
How many calories are in a single serving and the number of calories from fat in that serving. This is especially important for those who are cutting fat and calories to lose weight.

Use the Percent of Daily Values
Use the percent of Daily Values (DV) to help you evaluate how a particular food fits into your daily meal plan. Daily Values are average levels of nutrients for a person eating 2,000 calories a day. A food item with a 5% DV means 5% of the amount that a person consuming 2,000 calories a day would eat. Remember, the percent of DV is for the entire 2,000-calorie day, not just for one meal or snack. You may need more or less than 2,000 calories per day. For some nutrients, you may need more or less than the average DV.

High and Low of Daily Values
A DV of 5 percent or less is low. Try to aim low in total fat, saturated fat, cholesterol, and sodium. A DV of 20 percent or more is high. Try to aim high in vitamins, minerals and fiber.

Cut down Fat, Cholesterol and Sodium
Remember to aim low for the percent of DV of these nutrients. Eating less fat, cholesterol and sodium may help reduce your risk for heart disease, high blood pressure and cancer. Total fat includes saturated fat, polyunsaturated fat and monounsaturated fat. Limit total fat to 100% DV or less per day.

Saturated fat and trans fat are linked to an increased risk of heart disease. High levels of sodium can add up to high blood pressure.

Vitamins, Minerals & Fiber

Aim high for the percent of DV of these nutrients. Eat more fiber, vitamins A and C, calcium, and iron to maintain good health and help reduce your risk of certain health problems, such as osteoporosis and anemia. Choose more fruits and vegetables to get more of these nutrients.

Other Nutrients

Carbohydrates: There are three types of carbohydrates—sugars, starches and fiber.

Select whole-grain breads, cereals, rice and pasta plus fruits and vegetables.

Sugars: Simple carbohydrates or sugars occur naturally in foods such as fruit juice (fructose), or come from refined sources, such as table sugar (sucrose) or corn syrup.

Go over the Ingredient List

Foods with more than one ingredient must have an ingredient list on the label. Ingredients are listed in descending order by weight.
Ingredients in the largest amounts are listed first.
Manufacturers also are required to clearly state if food products may contain protein derived from the eight major allergenic foods.
These foods are milk, eggs, fish, crustacean shellfish, tree nuts, peanuts, wheat and soybeans.

Source: American Dietetic Association

Don't try to cut out all of these, your body needs these, but in moderation.

Learn your food pyramid, but don't be a fanatic about it.
Enjoy your food; don't cover it up with gravies & sauces.
Discover food all over again; learn to enjoy the taste of fresh
fruits, and vegetables, without adding things to them.

It's not rocket science, just good food science, and a little
common sense.

As for Meats:

This can be a hard subject for the male household members.
"You know the meat and potatoes thing"

Eat beef and pork in moderation, learn to enjoy poultry again.
Chicken & Turkey can be cooking in so many different way, that
when you discover all you can do with them you'll be surprising
your family with some amazing meals, like turkey spaghetti (in
recipe section)

Try this:
Break out the foreman Grill and start the grilling experience,
"I did & I love it."

You will be amazed at what you can make on this thing, and it's
so delicious too.

The fat drains off & the flavor is all that left behind.

So find yourself a good seasoning low in sodium and good to
use with meat as well as vegetables.

Sprinkle it on and grill away, vegetables turn out great and
meats turn out fantastic.

Just don't pour on things that add calories and fat.
Note: Try Worcestershire sauce instead of steak sauce and
ketchup.

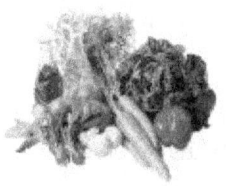

Now Breakfast can be a Challenge!!!!

Smoothies make a great breakfast, accompanied by a low-fat muffin.
Great with the kids too!
Smoothies Recipe in the Recipe Section

Try the Special K Challenge!

My favorite breakfast:
Now before you judge it, it's great tasting, and it keeps me full for 4 whole hours.
1 boiled egg (only eat the whites)
2 sliced of tomato
2 slices of deli style turkey ham
1 slice of whole wheat toast (you can even have cinnamon raisin bread)

Do your best to only eat the whites of the egg, all the fat and cholesterol is in the yoke.
Cut back on the coffee, if you're a coffee drinker.

Try your best to stay away from bacon, sausage, and grits, unless you use turkey products, and low sodium, low fat cheeses and margarine.

Limit your cheese to low fat cheese, or regular cheese in moderation, if at all.

Drink water, green tea or juice with your breakfast.

Another Breakfast of mine:
Using a ice cream scooper
3 scoops of low-fat yogurt (you can use flavored yogurt)
2/3 cup of special k w/berries
1 hand full of blueberries or strawberries, or
2 scoops of fruit cocktail
Buy your fruit fresh not frozen if possible
In a bowl, put your yogurt in, sprinkle the cereal over the yogurt and stir it up, top with your fruit.

Delicious!!!

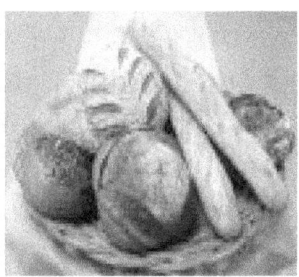

Now let's get into this Green Tea!

"Better to be deprived of food for three days, than tea for one."
(Ancient Chinese Proverb)

Green Tea and Weight Loss:
If you drink green tea you can-

- **Lower your cholesterol**
- **Increase thermo genesis (your body's calorie burning rate)**
- **Enhance fat oxidation**

The benefits of Green tea in weight loss- it burns fat naturally and increases metabolism

Green tea contains high concentrations of *catechin polyphenols. These compounds work with other chemicals to intensify levels of fat oxidation and thermo genesis, where heat is created in the body by burning fuels such as fat. Drinking green tea regularly will increase your metabolism and help burn fat safely and naturally.

I recommend quality teas based on their *catechin content, ease of preparation, and price.

*__Catechins__ *are powerful anti-oxidants. The best source of catechins is white tea, with green tea coming close. Catechins are believed to have some value in fighting tumors as well as enhancing immune system function. Other sources of catechins include dark chocolate and apples.*

Catechin is a tannin (**Tannin** is a large, astringent (meaning it tightens pores and draws liquids out)) particularly found in green and white tea because the black tea oxidation process reduces catechins in black tea. Catechin is a powerful, water soluble polyphenol and antioxidant that is easily oxidized. Several thousand types are available in the plant world. As many as two thousand are known to have a flavon structure and are called flavonoids. Catechin is one of them.

Expensive gourmet teas do the exact same thing Grocery green tea will do, so don't go out and buy the expensive one thinking it's better, NOT!!! Even if you have access to these, the ones you find in your local Health food store, Vitamin shops, grocery stores, and superstores will be fine.

Now to add my trick,
After I brew my green tea, and let it cool, I add light or diet apple, cranapple or cranberry juice to my tea instead of sugar or honey. Just ½ cup of juice to 1 cup of tea, you don't want to weaken your tea, just add a little flavor, and keep calories down. Enjoy!!!

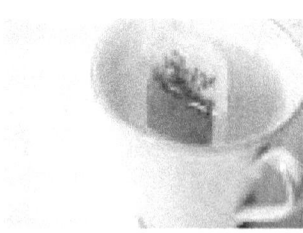

Let's Talk Lunch!

Lunch is Easy!

Make something light, like a platter salad for 2 or more.
(In the recipe section)

Smoothies are great for me; I get my fruit, and sometimes my vegetables too.

Fruit salads are wonderful, especially when the good fruits are in season like strawberries, and melons.

My favorite:

Yogurt Tart: (In the recipe section)

You can make these tarts ahead of time and keep them in a tight container, for snacking later, (very nutritious), and the kids just love them.

Tuna melts are divine: (In the recipe section)

Learn to make wrap-ups using your favorite healthy ingredients. Wrap them up in lettuce leaf or spinach & herb wrapper; them steam them on the countertop grill.

My favorite Wrap-up is in the recipe section.

Remember to drink plenty of water; you'll be surprised at the results from drinking 8-8oz of water a day. I know it sounds like a lot but if you think about it, babies drink 8oz bottles several times a day, if they can do it with their tiny stomachs, so can we.

Dinner Time!

Dinner can be a breeze!

Here is where that countertop grill comes in super handy!
"I believe I use mine everyday!
"Wouldn't be without it!"

Try:

Grilled Chicken Breast (discussed in the recipe section)
Tossed Salad
Green Tea

Just select things that appeal to your healthy side and cook it properly don't over cook, steam the vegetables.

Remember this: you don't have to stop eating the foods you love; you just need to learn to eat them in a healthier way.

You like steak, great, grill your steak and eat it just like that. Season it with a good Mrs. Dash seasoning, or seasoning salt call it done, no need for steak sauces, ketchup or gravies. That steak is great seasoned and grilled. Try it! "Don't Over Cook!"

Don't fry if you can help it.

I know that fried chicken sounds good tonight! But try this instead: Get some boneless chicken breast, and again season it with your favorite seasoning, and grill it up. "Don't Over Cook!"

Turkey burgers
(In the recipe section)

Bake, broil, or grill your meats, and experiment with your vegetables by grilling them as well, you'll be surprise at the taste.

Try to eliminate the fatty butters & margarine when flavoring your veggies. Use Mrs. Dash, Salt or Pepper.

Use low-fat dressings and don't load up your baked potato with sour cream, bacon, or gravies.
Use ICBINB and enjoy the natural delicious flavor of your food.

As always watch your sodium & fat intake with all your meals.

"I can't say it enough, Drink your water"

*ICBINB- I Can't Believe It's Not Butter

SNACKING!
Don't do it if you can help it!

This can be a huge problem for some people, especially during the late hours of the day.

Try the trail mix in the recipe section; it always gets me through the night when a snack attack comes my way. It's healthy, and the whole family just loves it. We leave it lying around in air tight containers all over the house, for snacking anytime.

Granola is good for snacking!
The tarts in the recipe section are great for snacking!
I eat Special K w/berries out of the box as a snack!
Cheerios are excellent and great for the heart!
Fresh fruit!
Eat Sherbet instead of ice cream!

Try not to make snacking a habit; you don't want to mess up what you've accomplished all day by snacking late night!

Healthy Food Shopping:

❖ Some of the foods on this list will not available to you until you start to train your body to except its new food habits.
❖ Fruit has to be limited in the beginning because of the natural fruit sugars; they can prohibit you from losing weight.

Fresh Vegetables

Lettuces	greens	cucumbers	carrots
Asparagus	zucchini	radishes	tomatoes
Green bean	onions	green onions	peppers
Cauliflower	broccoli	peas	celery
Potatoes "not too much"		corn	squash
Sweet Potatoes			

Notes:

_____

_____

Fresh fruits should be eaten in halves

Bananas	apples	oranges	pears
Peaches	nectarines	grapefruits	berries
*Strawberries	*Blueberries		

Notes: *are fruits that can be eaten as often as you like

_____

_____

Frozen Foods

Green beans	peas	mixed veg.	carrots
Chicken breast	fruit bars	shrimp	corn
Fish fillet "prefer fresh"		onions	turkey burgers

Notes:

_____

_____

Canned Foods

Black beans   tomatoes   marinara sauce   tuna
Salmon   beans   pinto beans "no pork"
Pineapples
Other Canned Foods: no salt canned veggies, and watch for pork in your bean products.
Notes:

_____

_____

Meats:

Ground turkey   turkey sausage   fish   salmon
Shell fish   chicken   tutkey

Notes:

_____

_____

Grains & Cereals

Whole wheat bread   Oatmeal   whole wheat pasta
Whole grain cereals

Notes:

_____

_____

Beverages

Water   Sparkling water   Water   Herb tea
Tomato juice   100 % fruit juice "not too much"

Notes:

_____

_____

Diary & Eggs

Low fat sour cream   low fat milk 2%   cheddar cheese
Low fat cream cheese   Colby cheese   mozzarella cheese
Non-fat or low fat yogurt

Notes:

_____

_____

Miscellaneous Items

Herb & spices   sesame oil   low fat dressings
Low fat mayonnaise   garlic   walnuts
Pumpkins seeds   mixed nuts   almonds
Pecans   mustard   EVOO "extra virgin olive oil"
Flax seeds   peanuts   low sodium soy sauce

*Water has to be your first choice when looking for something to quench your thirst. Your grocery store and/or superstores have a great selection of "On The Go" They don't add anything to your water but flavor.
Try it, it just might give you the help you need to get the amount of water intake you need on a daily basis.*

Notes:
- Get your green tea, and remember to mix it 2 parts tea to 1 part juice, don't use sugar or honey in your tea
- Watch your Sodium and Fats
- Exercise, even it's it just walking
- Get adequate sleep nightly, You body has to rest & rejuvenate
- Drink plenty of water 8-8oz glasses a day,
- **"YOU CAN DO IT!"**
- Make sure you eat a good supply of fiber daily, Elimination is the key to good weight loss
- A trick I learned, bathe daily, showers are good, but your body expels waste through your pore too, so soaking in a hot bath with non- clogging soaps, bubble bath, and gels with help aid in the weight loss.

The Importance of Water

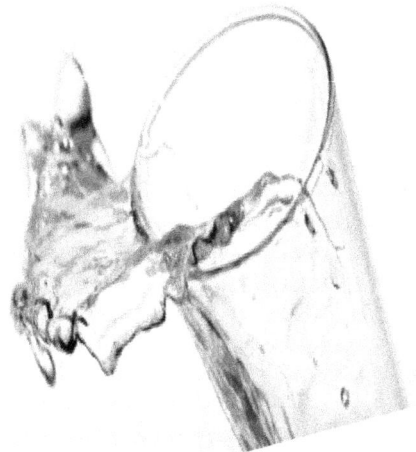

There are a few things that we cannot ignore to sustain a good and a healthy life. The main things that we should take care of to have a good health are diet, sleep and exercise.

No matter how good you eat, if you don't sleep well and don't exercise, there will be problems.

- If you exercise, but don't eat healthy and get the proper rest you're still out of balance, and you won't be benefited.

- **The main rule to lead a healthy life is the right diet,**
  The right amount of sleep and the correct proportion of exercise. These are the key ingredients that make up good health.

- Most of us know the importance of a good diet. But it's just as important to have the equal right amount of water, in direct or indirect form.

- There are countless benefits of consuming water.
  Water makes up a large part of our body.
  Most of our body weight is due to the bones and the water contained in our body.

If you don't drink water in the right quantity you may face certain problems.

- Water is known to be like a solvent in the body "very valuable"
Hence it can easily dissolve any toxic material present in our body. The right amount of water is absolutely essential to keep the salts in our body in a non toxic form. The water helps us keep the salt present in our body in a non toxic form.
If you do not consume the right amount of water in your diet, the salt that is deposited under the skin is converted into a toxic form and can lead to problems.

- The other important use of water is that it helps us remove the dirt and other toxics from our body.

  People, who don't drink the necessary amount of water, face the problems like acne, etc.

- The right amount of water in the diet also keeps the skin moisturized.

  If the amount of water you drink is less than the amount required by the body, it may lead to dry, crack skin.

  Another important factor of drinking the right amount of water in our diet is that if you don't consume the right amount of water, you may face the problems of dehydration, and you may have to be hospitalized.

  You should consume at least two liters of water each day, to have a good health, and to prevent the problems associated with the lack of water.

- Action steps
Drink at least two liters of water everyday, to maintain the right amount of water (8-8oz glasses)
Water should be avoided directly after the meals. You may drink water, during the meal or before it.

The Benefits of Apple Cider Vinegar

Apple Cider Vinegar has been used as a health aid for thousands of years. For many of us it is a common item on our grocery list and with good reason.

It's rich in vitamins and minerals as well as enzymes, amino acids, potash, prop ionic acid and apple pectin.

It can lower cholesterol by flushing fats, thins blood to help control blood pressure and its fiber helps to control glucose in the blood.

While we are told to stay away from vinegar if we have a yeast infection, **organic** apple cider vinegar aids in stopping the infection.

Apple cider vinegar has a powerful detoxifying and purifying influence and has been known for its ability to neutralize harmful bacteria that may be found in foods. By taking a tablespoon in a glass of water before a meal, it could prevent upset stomach or diarrhea.

Its said to be beneficial in the treatment of arthritis, bladder problems, metabolism, sore throats, gallstones, kidney stones, stiff joints, detoxifying the body, weight loss, and is taken regularly for all over good health.

Apple Cider Vinegar can be taken three times a day by mixing 1 or 2 tablespoons of vinegar in 8 ounces of distilled water, and honey to taste "not too much guys".

Always drink Apple cider vinegar diluted.

Use a straw or rinse your mouth with water directly after drinking to avoid enamel erosion on teeth.

You should always consult your doctor before making changes to your treatment

Too Much Fruit Can Be Bad

Many of us have come to believe that eating healthier means eating lots of fruits and vegetables.

While fruits and vegetables are much better for you than refined foods like cookies and chips, my experience has led me to believe that too much fruit can be harmful to your diet.

A lot of the fruit that is grown today is much higher in sugar.

Have you ever tasted a wild blueberry?
How about a wild apple?

On their own, they are delicious, but you may be surprised to discover that they aren't nearly as sweet as modern day varieties.

Try Organic!

Watch out for Hybrid fruits, they carry way more sugar then you need!

But sugar from fruit is all natural, so you should be able to eat as much as you want, right?

Have you ever heard of a fruitarian?
Fruitarians are people who eat nothing but raw fruits.

It is not uncommon for a strict fruitarian to eat five bananas and five dates for breakfast, one large cantaloupe for lunch, and five large peaches for dinner.

Some fruitarians take a more balanced approach and eat lots of less sweet, seed-bearing fruits like tomatoes and zucchini. They also eat plenty of greens like romaine lettuce.

Regardless of which approach is taken, strict fruitarian of more than two years who didn't have significant health challenges.

The most common challenges:

Dental decay
Osteoporosis
Wasting of muscle tissue
Inability to maintain a healthy weight
Chronic fatigue
Skin problems
Thinning hair
Weakening nails
Excessive irritability

Some of these problems are the result of nutritional deficiency. The most common deficiencies in the world today are:
Vitamin B12
Vitamin A
Vitamin D
Zinc
Certain essential fatty acids

Problems with a high fruit diet is that it can lead to problems involving the hormones that regulate your blood sugar; insulin, glucagon, and growth hormone.

Chronic imbalance of these hormones is a sure way to develop cardiovascular disease and diabetes.

The good news is that when you eat fruits in moderately, they can contribute to excellent overall health and fitness.

Here is a list of some of my favorite, healthy fruits:

1. **Berries** - Be sure that they are wild or organic, as commercially grown berries are heavily coated with pesticides. Berries tend to put less stress on your blood sugar - regulating mechanisms than other fruits, and provide loads of fiber, vitamins, and minerals, which protect you against disease. Frozen wild blueberries are available year-round in almost any grocery store.

2. **Avocado** - An excellent source of raw fat, which is essential for healing and maintenance of health. Avocados are also an excellent source of fiber, vitamins, and minerals. The fatty acids found in avocados provide excellent fuel for energy. A good avocado has a rich, creamy texture and a rich green color towards the outer part of its flesh.

3. **Figs** - If you haven't tried a fresh black or green fig, you are missing out on one of the most mineral full and dense fruits there is. Fresh figs are superior to dried figs, as the drying process creates an unhealthy concentration of the natural sugars in figs. If you are going to eat dried figs, strive to eat only a few per day. Figs are particularly high in potassium, calcium, and iron.

4. **Pomegranates** – Are my favorite fruit, and a super antioxidant. If you could choose only one fruit to get into your blood and provide great protection against free radical damage and chronic disease, pomegranates would be a great choice. By weight, they have one of the highest concentrated antioxidant among all fruits.

5. **Apples** - Are high in fiber, vitamins, minerals, and antioxidants. They are the most affordable fruits to eat on a regular basis.

If you want to eat sweet fruit like bananas, grapes, and ripe persimmons, you need to eat half of it or you may eat them with some dark green foods like lettuce, celery sticks, and avocado, as the mineral density in these green foods will help to dampen the unhealthy effect that sweet fruits have on your insulin levels.

Try to limit your fruit juices intake, as their concentrated sugars contribute to health problems related to too much insulin production.

The Food Pyramid

Get to know the pyramid; it will help you to plan your meals, and snacks for your family.

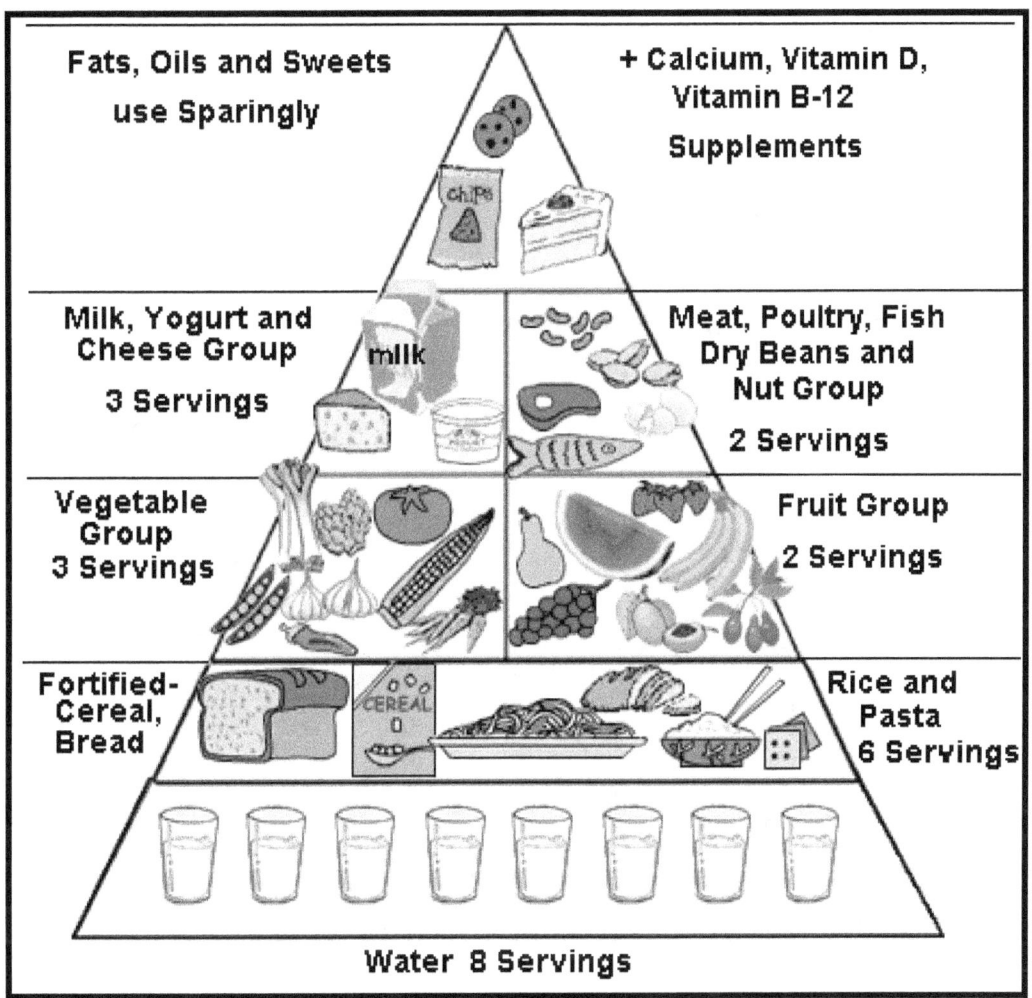

Exercise:
Exercise doesn't have to be difficult, a long ordeal, or feared. You can start with walking in your neighborhood, parking the car a little further out then normal in parking lots, become a mall walker, etc.
Join the YMCA
Sign up for am aerobics class
Buy DVD exercise videos if you prefer the privacy of your own home.
"Just Exercise!"

Recipe Section

- Smoothie

3 scoops of low fat yogurt
½ cup of orange juice
½ cups of fresh fruit
2 cups of ice

Cut your fruit into chunks,
Always measure you juice
Add the yogurt tot the mixer first
Then the ice, fruit and juice
Blend in your smoothie maker or blender and enjoy!

- Wrap-ups

2-3 strips of grilled chicken breasts
2 strips of avocado
1 tsp of bean sprouts
1 tsp of corn

On a wonton wrapper: arrange all your ingredients, and follow the directions on the package on how to tuck and roll up your wrapper, and fry in smart balance oil under golden brown.

In a lettuce leaf: arrange all your ingredients and rolls up, pick toothpicks in the roll to help hold it shape. Place in a streamer few a couple of minutes to warm, or place in the microwave it for 30 seconds.

- Platter Salad

Tuna	Boiled eggs (whites only)
Claw meat crab	Cucumbers
Lettuce	Carrots
Tomato wedges	Mushroom
Avocado Slices	Grapes
Crackers	
Low-fat dressings	

On a large platter, garnish the whole bottom of the platter with lettuce, starting in the center of the platter, place your egg whites in a circular mound, then go around them with your tomato wedges, then your carrots, and so on until you use all your ingredients. The tuna and the crab should always be the last thing on the platter as not to lend their smell to the other foods.

Serve your cracker on a separate dish or on the edge on the platter.
Have light dressing to accompany.
Serve with your delicious Green Tea & Juice Mixture.

- Trail Mix

Cashews
Lots of Raisins
Sunflower seeds (shelled)
Pumpkin seeds (shelled)
Dried cranberries

Just mix everything together and storage in air tight containers all over the house. The kids will love it, I do!

- Tuna Melt

2 slices of whole wheat toast buttered with ICBINB
Tuna packed in water (always)
Salt & pepper
Mrs. Dash (Your choice & optional)
1 slice of low fat mozzarella cheese
1 slice of low fat cheddar cheese

Make your toast and spread some ICBINB on it, Break up
your tuna, and season with salt, pepper, and Mrs. Dash.
Place the mozzarella cheese on your toast and top with the
tuna mixture, then top with the cheddar cheese and top with
the other slice of toast.
Microwave for 30 seconds or until cheese melts or even
better
Place in the oven on 350 until cheese melts.
Delicious, and look at how many calories you saved.

- Tart

4 cups of Special K w/ berries or Total
½ cups of apple juice
A sprinkle of cinnamon
2 eggs whites

In a bowl put all your cereal in, beat the cinnamon, egg
whites and the juice together, and pour over the cereal, mix it
all up until each piece of cereal is coated and moist. Press
into a round greased cake pan, make sure it's all evened out,
and bake for 10-12 minutes.   Yummy!!!

- Shepherd's Pie

1½ lbs of lean ground turkey
2 packages of instant mashed potatoes
1 can of green peas
1 package of low-fat shredded cheddar cheese

Make you mashed potatoes the normal way and set aside,
Ground your ground turkey, and drain off the fat, remember
to use smart balance oil.
Drain your peas.
Now in an ungreased baking pan, spoon in a layer of meat,
top with a layer of peas, and layer of mashed potatoes, if you
like you can make as many layers as you like or just one of
each.
Top it off with the shredded cheese and bake and the cheese
is brown.

- Grilled Chicken, "a no brainer"
Just whip out the countertop grill and go to work,
Remember not to add anything that will add calories to your
meat.
Just season and grill.

** Turkey Burgers
 (4 servings)

4 turkey burgers (you can find them in the frozen meat section)
1 medium onion
1 large tomato
1 teaspoon of minced garlic
Grill seasoning
A-1 steak sauce & water

Heat a skillet over medium heat.
Add a tablespoon of smart balance spread.
Separate the burgers carefully, they are delicate.
Season them with the grill seasoning, and place in the skillet, seasoning side down, now season the other side. Do the same with the remaining burgers, add the garlic and cover for about 2 minute while you chop up the onion, and tomato.

Set them aside and check on your burgers, it's time to turn them over.
Now add the onion, tomato, and A-1 sauce, cover and let simmer.
Cook over low heat, checking and turning to prevent sticking, add water to keep moist and to help create the gravy.

Cook until the vegetables are tender, and the gravy is to your liking.
Serve with plain rice or other vegetables.

**Turkey Spaghetti

1 roll of ground turkey
1 roll of turkey breakfast sausage
1 box of whole grain spaghetti
2 shallots diced
1 large onion diced
1 green pepper diced
2 tablespoon of garlic
1 can of diced tomatoes drained
1 can of garlic & herb spaghetti sauce
½ can of traditional spaghetti sauce
Original Ms Dash
Salt & Pepper
Italian seasoning
EVOO- extra virgin olive oil

In your first dutch oven pot add water until you half way fill the pot, add a little EVOO to prevent the pasta from sticking, and bring to a boil.

Heat the other dutch oven over medium high heat, add 2 tbsp of EVOO
While waiting for the oil to heat make sure you have all your vegetables diced up.
Crumble the ground turkey into the pot, followed by the turkey sausage and garlic, stirring constantly to prevent sticking, now add your Ms Dash to taste along with the Italian seasoning.
Cook over medium heat until almost brown.
Drain off any left over oil, and start adding your vegetables one at a time, shallots first, onions, green peppers, leaving the diced tomatoes for last.
Continue to simmer over medium low heat until the vegetables are tender, then add the tomatoes, and fold in the mixture.
Add the remaining ingredients, and simmer over low heat while you wait for the pasta to cook.
Serve however you like, mixed together or sauce served on top of a bed of pasta.
Enjoy!

- Basil Tomatoes, and Fresh Mozzarella

  4 tomatoes, each cut into 6 slices (about 1 1/2 pounds)
  1/2 pound fresh mozzarella cheese, cut into 12 slices
  1/4 teaspoon kosher salt
  1/4 teaspoon freshly ground black pepper
  1 tablespoon extra virgin olive oil
  1/2 cup fresh basil leaves

  Arrange 4 tomato slices and 2 mozzarella slices on each of 6 salad plates. Sprinkle evenly with salt and pepper; drizzle with oil. Top evenly with basil.

- Turkey meatloaf

  1 pound 93%-lean ground turkey
  1 medium zucchini, shredded
  1 cup finely chopped onion
  1 cup finely chopped red bell pepper
  1/3 cup uncooked whole-wheat couscous
  1 large egg, lightly beaten
  2 tablespoons Worcestershire sauce
  1 tablespoon Dijon mustard
  1/2 teaspoon freshly ground pepper
  1/4 teaspoon salt
  1/4 cup A-1 sauce (optional)

  Preheat oven to 400 degrees F. spray a pan with cooking spray.

  Mix turkey, couscous, zucchini, onion, bell pepper, egg, Worcestershire, mustard, pepper and salt in a large bowl. Place in the pan and mold into a loaf, spread A-1 on top of loaf

  Bake until the meatloaf is cooked through or an instant-read thermometer inserted into the center registers 165 degrees F, about 25 minutes. Let the loaf stand in the pan for 5 minutes before serving.

Natural Appetite Suppressants

Apples
An apple a day helps with cravings.
High-fiber foods like apples generally require more chewing time, giving your body extra time to register the fact that you're no longer hungry.
Therefore, you're less likely to overeat.
Apples are also a natural anti-inflammatory.

Pine Nuts
Pine nuts contain the highest amount of protein of any nut or seed.
You can take a handful of pine nuts with a meal to create a feeling of fullness.
How you ask?
Pine nuts contain *pinolenic acid, a naturally occurring polyunsaturated fat that stimulates two powerful hunger suppressing hormones.
Both hormones play a major role in signaling to the brain that you're no longer hungry

*Pinolenic Acid, a natural plant extract, can provide a feeling of fullness, thereby reducing the amount of food you consume.

Benefits of Pinolenic Acid

- Reduces serum insulin production to prohibit the buildup of fat cells
- Decreased risk of DNA damage from insulin overload
- Helps prevent obesity and related health problems
- Aids in digestion and boosts stamina to encourage calorie burning
- Promotes "satiety" (a sense of fullness) to combat the desire to eat
- Works to lower blood sugar and cholesterol levels

Flaxseeds

Flaxseed oil is the best known source of omega-3 fats but raw flaxseeds are even better, especially for appetite control.
One ounce of flaxseed provides the added benefit of 8 grams of fiber.
The more fiber you eat at any meal or snack, the slower your blood sugar, helping to control the hunger hormones.
Flaxseeds go good in salads, smoothies or sprinkled over vegetables and yogurt.
Flaxseeds have cancer preventive properties and lowers cholesterol.

Oatmeal

Real oatmeal -- not instant -- is the healthiest of all carbohydrates. It's low on the glycemic load scale and has high fiber content, when it enters bloodstream it slow and keeps you feeling full for a long time.
One bowl of oatmeal consumed daily can reduce cholesterol.
For breakfast or as a snack, a small bowl makes an excellent hunger reducer. Try adding a little light buttery spread or a handful of pine nuts for longer-lasting fullness. Or how about sprinkling on some ground flaxseed or cinnamon?

Salad

To avoid overeating, try eating a small salad before a meal.
The fiber helps slow the entrance of glucose (sugar) into the bloodstream, making you less likely to be hungry.
Try varying your salad choices with spinach, endives and cabbages -- all types of greens will help curb your cravings.

Soup

Soup is a great way to tone down or control the appetite and the secret is soup's combination of high water and low calories. Make sure to choose broths or vegetable soups, not the creamy-rich ones.

Go Green Tea

If you drink a bottle of tea fortified with green tea extract (GTE) every day for three months you could lose more body fat than people who drink tea without GTE. To get the benefits, researchers suggest drinking several cups of green tea each day.

Think Small

Using small salad plates and bowls can help you eat 30 percent fewer calories at meals. Not to mention you should drink out of skinny glasses (versus short, wide glasses), and you'll serve yourself 28 percent less.

Eat Grapefruits

It's no myth: Grapefruits are a great weight loss aid. People who ate half a grapefruit three times a day (before each meal) lost an average of 3.6 pounds. Grapefruits may lower insulin, a fat storage hormone.

Sleep, Sleep and more Sleep

Women that sleep less than seven hours a night put on more weight during middle age than women who sleep more.
This is the time of day that your body is most vulnerable, your resistance is lower in the evenings hours, and needs rest to rejuvenate.
Rest, Rest, and more Rest
Rest, water, a good diet and exercise is a routine you can be proud of.

Affirmations

Affirmations are testimonials of approval that you use to allow the signs of your destiny.

They are meaningful and positive statements sent out to the universe.

To have positive affirmations, you need to eliminate the negativity around you.

You must first believe that you can create your own destiny.

Maybe, or I'll try is not allowed here.

Positive is how you live for now on.

Affirmations for Health

- I have the authority to control my health.
- I am in control of my health and well being.
- I have plenty of energy, vitality and well-being.
- I am healthy in all facets of my being.
- I don't fear being unhealthy because I know that I have control of my own body.
- I am capable of maintaining an ideal weight.
- I possess the energy I need to do all the daily activities in my life.
- My mind is free and at peace.
- I love and care for my body and it cares for me.

My Affirmations

"I am aware of how great I am, that's why I have no boundaries
My resources are great, my abilities are great, my potential is
great"

"I am aware of how great I am, that's why I have no boundaries
My resources are great, my abilities are great, my potential is
great"

"I am aware of how great I am, that's why I have no boundaries
My resources are great, my abilities are great, my potential is
great"

"My thoughts, my words, my actions really create who I am.
That is why I think Positively, I say positive words, and I take
positive actions."

"My thoughts, my words, my actions really create who I am.
That is why I think Positively, I say positive words, and I take
positive actions."

"My thoughts, my words, my actions really create who I am.
That is why I think Positively, I say positive words, and I take
positive actions."

"My thoughts, my words, my actions really create who I am.
That is why I think Positively, I say positive words, and I take
positive actions."

"The people I need to meet will always come my way."
"The people I need to meet will always come my way."
"The people I need to meet will always come my way."
"The people I need to meet will always come my way."
"The people I need to meet will always come my way."
"The people I need to meet will always come my way."

"I know what my Blessings feel like. I know what they smell like and taste like.
I envision my life Blessed, and fulfilled as the Lord intended for me."

"I know what my Blessings feel like. I know what they smell like and taste like.
I envision my life Blessed, and fulfilled as the Lord intended for me."

"I know what my Blessings feel like. I know what they smell like and taste like.
I envision my life Blessed, and fulfilled as the Lord intended for me."

"I know what my Blessings feel like. I know what they smell like and taste like.
I envision my life Blessed, and fulfilled as the Lord intended for me."

Make Your Own Affirmations:

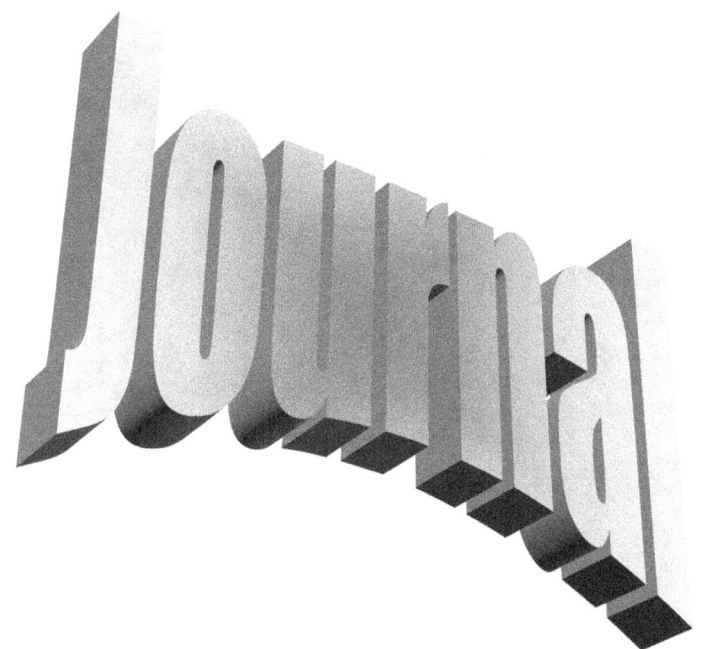

Journal

_____
_____
_____
_____
_____
_____
_____
_____
_____
_____
_____
_____
_____
_____
_____
_____
_____
_____
_____
_____
_____
_____
_____
_____
_____
_____
_____
_____
_____
_____
_____
_____
_____
_____
_____
_____

Journal

Journal

Journal

Journal

Journal

Journal

_____
_____
_____
_____
_____
_____
_____
_____
_____
_____
_____
_____
_____
_____
_____
_____
_____
_____
_____
_____
_____
_____
_____
_____
_____
_____
_____
_____
_____
_____
_____
_____
_____
_____
_____
_____
_____

Journal

Journal

_____
_____
_____
_____
_____
_____
_____
_____
_____
_____
_____
_____
_____
_____
_____
_____
_____
_____
_____
_____
_____
_____
_____
_____
_____
_____
_____
_____
_____
_____
_____
_____
_____
_____
_____
_____

Journal

_____
_____
_____
_____
_____
_____
_____
_____
_____
_____
_____
_____
_____
_____
_____
_____
_____
_____
_____
_____
_____
_____
_____
_____
_____
_____
_____
_____
_____
_____
_____
_____

Journal

_____
_____
_____
_____
_____
_____
_____
_____
_____
_____
_____
_____
_____
_____
_____
_____
_____
_____
_____
_____
_____
_____
_____
_____
_____
_____
_____
_____
_____
_____
_____
_____
_____
_____
_____

Journal

Journal

Journal

Journal

Journal

_____
_____
_____
_____
_____
_____
_____
_____
_____
_____
_____
_____
_____
_____
_____
_____
_____
_____
_____
_____
_____
_____
_____
_____
_____
_____
_____
_____
_____
_____
_____
_____
_____
_____
_____
_____
_____

Journal

Journal

Journal

Journal

Journal

Journal

Journal

_____
_____
_____
_____
_____
_____
_____
_____
_____
_____
_____
_____
_____
_____
_____
_____
_____
_____
_____
_____
_____
_____
_____
_____
_____
_____
_____
_____
_____
_____
_____
_____

Journal

Journal

Journal

Journal

Journal

Journal

Journal

Journal

Journal

_____
_____
_____
_____
_____
_____
_____
_____
_____
_____
_____
_____
_____
_____
_____
_____
_____
_____
_____
_____
_____
_____
_____
_____
_____
_____
_____
_____
_____
_____
_____
_____
_____
_____
_____

Journal

Journal

_____
_____
_____
_____
_____
_____
_____
_____
_____
_____
_____
_____
_____
_____
_____
_____
_____
_____
_____
_____
_____
_____
_____
_____
_____
_____
_____
_____
_____
_____
_____
_____
_____
_____

Journal

Journal

Journal

Journal

Journal

Journal

Journal

_____
_____
_____
_____
_____
_____
_____
_____
_____
_____
_____
_____
_____
_____
_____
_____
_____
_____
_____
_____
_____
_____
_____
_____
_____
_____
_____
_____
_____
_____
_____
_____

Journal

Journal

_____
_____
_____
_____
_____
_____
_____
_____
_____
_____
_____
_____
_____
_____
_____
_____
_____
_____
_____
_____
_____
_____
_____
_____
_____
_____
_____
_____
_____
_____
_____
_____
_____
_____
_____

Journal

Journal

Journal

Journal

Weight Tracker

Weight Loss Tracker

Day: _____

Goal: _____

Weight: _____

Achievement:

_____
_____
_____
_____
_____
_____

Day: _____

Goal: _____

Weight: _____

Achievement:

_____
_____
_____
_____
_____

Day: _____

Goal: _____

Weight: _____

Achievement:

_____
_____
_____
_____
_____
_____

Weight Loss Tracker

Day: _____

Goal: _____

Weight: _____

Achievement:

_____
_____
_____
_____
_____

Day: _____

Goal: _____

Weight: _____

Achievement:

_____
_____
_____
_____
_____

Day: _____

Goal: _____

Weight: _____

Achievement:

_____
_____
_____
_____
_____

Weight Loss Tracker

Day: _____

Goal: _____

Weight: _____

Achievement:

_____
_____
_____
_____
_____

Day: _____

Goal: _____

Weight: _____

Achievement:

_____
_____
_____
_____
_____

Day: _____

Goal: _____

Weight: _____

Achievement:

_____
_____
_____
_____
_____

Weight Loss Tracker

Day: _____

Goal: _____

Weight: _____

Achievement:

_____
_____
_____
_____
_____

Day: _____

Goal: _____

Weight: _____

Achievement:

_____
_____
_____
_____
_____

Day: _____

Goal: _____

Weight: _____

Achievement:

_____
_____
_____
_____
_____

Weight Loss Tracker

Day: _____

Goal: _____

Weight: _____

Achievement:

_____

_____

_____

_____

_____

Day: _____

Goal: _____

Weight: _____

Achievement:

_____

_____

_____

_____

_____

Day: _____

Goal: _____

Weight: _____

Achievement:

_____

_____

_____

_____

_____

_____

Weight Loss Tracker

Day: _____

Goal: _____

Weight: _____

Achievement:

_____
_____
_____
_____
_____

Day: _____

Goal: _____

Weight: _____

Achievement:

_____
_____
_____
_____
_____

Day: _____

Goal: _____

Weight: _____

Achievement:

_____
_____
_____
_____
_____
_____

Weight Loss Tracker

Day: _____

Goal: _____

Weight: _____

Achievement:

_____
_____
_____
_____
_____

Day: _____

Goal: _____

Weight: _____

Achievement:

_____
_____
_____
_____
_____

Day: _____

Goal: _____

Weight: _____

Achievement:

_____
_____
_____
_____
_____
_____

Weight Loss Tracker

Day: _____
Goal: _____
Weight: _____

Achievement:

_____
_____
_____
_____
_____

Day: _____
Goal: _____
Weight: _____

Achievement:

_____
_____
_____
_____
_____

Day: _____
Goal: _____
Weight: _____

Achievement:

_____
_____
_____
_____
_____

Weight Loss Tracker

Day: _____

Goal: _____

Weight: _____

Achievement:

_____

_____

_____

_____

_____

Day: _____

Goal: _____

Weight: _____

Achievement:

_____

_____

_____

_____

_____

Day: _____

Goal: _____

Weight: _____

Achievement:

_____

_____

_____

_____

_____

_____

Weight Loss Tracker

Day: _____

Goal: _____

Weight: _____

Achievement:

_____

_____

_____

_____

_____

Day: _____

Goal: _____

Weight: _____

Achievement:

_____

_____

_____

_____

_____

Day: _____

Goal: _____

Weight: _____

Achievement:

_____

_____

_____

_____

_____

Weight Loss Tracker

Day: _____

Goal: _____

Weight: _____

Achievement:

_____

_____

_____

_____

_____

Day: _____

Goal: _____

Weight: _____

Achievement:

_____

_____

_____

_____

_____

Day: _____

Goal: _____

Weight: _____

Achievement:

_____

_____

_____

_____

_____

Weight Loss Tracker

Day: _____

Goal: _____

Weight: _____

Achievement:

_____
_____
_____
_____
_____

Day: _____

Goal: _____

Weight: _____

Achievement:

_____
_____
_____
_____
_____

Day: _____

Goal: _____

Weight: _____

Achievement:

_____
_____
_____
_____
_____

Weight Loss Tracker

Day: _____

Goal: _____

Weight: _____

Achievement:

_____

_____

_____

_____

_____

_____

Day: _____

Goal: _____

Weight: _____

Achievement:

_____

_____

_____

_____

_____

_____

Day: _____

Goal: _____

Weight: _____

Achievement:

_____

_____

_____

_____

_____

_____

Weight Loss Tracker

Day: _____

Goal: _____

Weight: _____

Achievement:

_____
_____
_____
_____
_____

Day: _____

Goal: _____

Weight: _____

Achievement:

_____
_____
_____
_____
_____

Day: _____

Goal: _____

Weight: _____

Achievement:

_____
_____
_____
_____
_____

Weight Loss Tracker

Day: _____

Goal: _____

Weight: _____

Achievement:

_____

_____

_____

_____

_____

Day: _____

Goal: _____

Weight: _____

Achievement:

_____

_____

_____

_____

_____

Day: _____

Goal: _____

Weight: _____

Achievement:

_____

_____

_____

_____

_____

_____

Weight Loss Tracker

Day: _____

Goal: _____

Weight: _____

Achievement:

_____

_____

_____

_____

_____

Day: _____

Goal: _____

Weight: _____

Achievement:

_____

_____

_____

_____

_____

Day: _____

Goal: _____

Weight: _____

Achievement:

_____

_____

_____

_____

_____

_____

Weight Loss Tracker

Day: _____

Goal: _____

Weight: _____

Achievement:

_____

_____

_____

_____

_____

Day: _____

Goal: _____

Weight: _____

Achievement:

_____

_____

_____

_____

_____

Day: _____

Goal: _____

Weight: _____

Achievement:

_____

_____

_____

_____

_____

Weight Loss Tracker

Day: _____

Goal: _____

Weight: _____

Achievement:

_____
_____
_____
_____
_____

Day: _____

Goal: _____

Weight: _____

Achievement:

_____
_____
_____
_____
_____

Day: _____

Goal: _____

Weight: _____

Achievement:

_____
_____
_____
_____
_____

Weight Loss Tracker

Day: _____

Goal: _____

Weight: _____

Achievement:

_____
_____
_____
_____
_____

Day: _____

Goal: _____

Weight: _____

Achievement:

_____
_____
_____
_____
_____

Day: _____

Goal: _____

Weight: _____

Achievement:

_____
_____
_____
_____
_____

Weight Loss Tracker

Day: _____

Goal: _____

Weight: _____

Achievement:

_____
_____
_____
_____
_____

Day: _____

Goal: _____

Weight: _____

Achievement:

_____
_____
_____
_____
_____

Day: _____

Goal: _____

Weight: _____

Achievement:

_____
_____
_____
_____
_____

Weight Loss Tracker

Day: _____

Goal: _____

Weight: _____

Achievement:

_____

_____

_____

_____

_____

Day: _____

Goal: _____

Weight: _____

Achievement:

_____

_____

_____

_____

_____

Day: _____

Goal: _____

Weight: _____

Achievement:

_____

_____

_____

_____

_____

Weight Loss Tracker

Day: _____

Goal: _____

Weight: _____

Achievement:

_____

_____

_____

_____

_____

Day: _____

Goal: _____

Weight: _____

Achievement:

_____

_____

_____

_____

_____

Day: _____

Goal: _____

Weight: _____

Achievement:

_____

_____

_____

_____

_____

_____

Weight Loss Tracker

Day: _____

Goal: _____

Weight: _____

Achievement:

_____

_____

_____

_____

_____

Day: _____

Goal: _____

Weight: _____

Achievement:

_____

_____

_____

_____

_____

Day: _____

Goal: _____

Weight: _____

Achievement:

_____

_____

_____

_____

_____

Weight Loss Tracker

Day: _____

Goal: _____

Weight: _____

Achievement:

_____
_____
_____
_____
_____

Day: _____

Goal: _____

Weight: _____

Achievement:

_____
_____
_____
_____
_____

Day: _____

Goal: _____

Weight: _____

Achievement:

_____
_____
_____
_____
_____

Weight Loss Tracker

Day: _____

Goal: _____

Weight: _____

Achievement:

_____

_____

_____

_____

_____

Day: _____

Goal: _____

Weight: _____

Achievement:

_____

_____

_____

_____

_____

Day: _____

Goal: _____

Weight: _____

Achievement:

_____

_____

_____

_____

_____

_____

Weight Loss Tracker

Day: _____
Goal: _____
Weight: _____

Achievement:

_____
_____
_____
_____
_____

Day: _____
Goal: _____
Weight: _____

Achievement:

_____
_____
_____
_____
_____

Day: _____
Goal: _____
Weight: _____

Achievement:

_____
_____
_____
_____
_____

Weight Loss Tracker

Day: _____

Goal: _____

Weight: _____

Achievement:

_____

_____

_____

_____

_____

Day: _____

Goal: _____

Weight: _____

Achievement:

_____

_____

_____

_____

_____

Day: _____

Goal: _____

Weight: _____

Achievement:

_____

_____

_____

_____

_____

Weight Loss Tracker

Day: _____

Goal: _____

Weight: _____

Achievement:

_____

_____

_____

_____

_____

Day: _____

Goal: _____

Weight: _____

Achievement:

_____

_____

_____

_____

_____

Day: _____

Goal: _____

Weight: _____

Achievement:

_____

_____

_____

_____

_____

_____

Weight Loss Tracker

Day: _____

Goal: _____

Weight: _____

Achievement:

_____

_____

_____

_____

_____

Day: _____

Goal: _____

Weight: _____

Achievement:

_____

_____

_____

_____

_____

Day: _____

Goal: _____

Weight: _____

Achievement:

_____

_____

_____

_____

_____

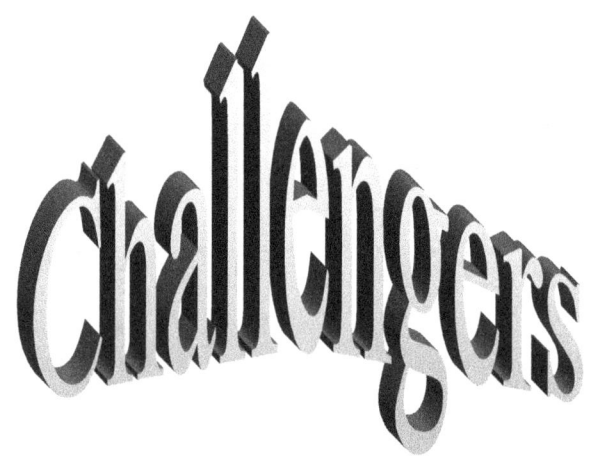

Challengers

Name: _____
Phone: _____
Notes:

_____
_____
_____
_____

Name: _____
Phone: _____
Notes:

_____
_____
_____
_____

Name: _____
Phone: _____
Notes:

_____
_____
_____
_____

Name: _____
Phone: _____
Notes:

_____
_____
_____
_____

Name: _____
Phone: _____
Notes:

_____
_____
_____
_____

Challengers

Name: _____
Phone: _____
Notes:

_____
_____
_____
_____
_____

Name: _____
Phone: _____
Notes:

_____
_____
_____
_____
_____

Name: _____
Phone: _____
Notes:

_____
_____
_____
_____
_____

Name: _____
Phone: _____
Notes:

_____
_____
_____
_____

Name: _____
Phone: _____
Notes:

_____
_____
_____
_____

Challengers

Name: _____
Phone: _____
Notes:

_____
_____
_____
_____

Name: _____
Phone: _____
Notes:

_____
_____
_____
_____

Name: _____
Phone: _____
Notes:

_____
_____
_____
_____

Name: _____
Phone: _____
Notes:

_____
_____
_____
_____

Name: _____
Phone: _____
Notes:

_____
_____
_____
_____

Challengers

Name: _____
Phone: _____
Notes:

_____
_____
_____
_____

Name: _____
Phone: _____
Notes:

_____
_____
_____
_____

Name: _____
Phone: _____
Notes:

_____
_____
_____
_____

Name: _____
Phone: _____
Notes:

_____
_____
_____
_____

Name: _____
Phone: _____
Notes:

_____
_____
_____
_____

Challengers

Name: _____
Phone: _____
Notes:

_____
_____
_____
_____

Name: _____
Phone: _____
Notes:

_____
_____
_____
_____

Name: _____
Phone: _____
Notes:

_____
_____
_____
_____

Name: _____
Phone: _____
Notes:

_____
_____
_____
_____

Name: _____
Phone: _____
Notes:

_____
_____
_____
_____

Challengers

Name: _____

Phone: _____

Notes:

_____

_____

_____

_____

Name: _____

Phone: _____

Notes:

_____

_____

_____

_____

Name: _____

Phone: _____

Notes:

_____

_____

_____

_____

Name: _____

Phone: _____

Notes:

_____

_____

_____

_____

Name: _____

Phone: _____

Notes:

_____

_____

_____

_____

Challengers

Name: _____
Phone: _____
Notes:

_____
_____
_____
_____

Name: _____
Phone: _____
Notes:

_____
_____
_____
_____

Name: _____
Phone: _____
Notes:

_____
_____
_____
_____

Name: _____
Phone: _____
Notes:

_____
_____
_____
_____

Name: _____
Phone: _____
Notes:

_____
_____
_____
_____

Challengers

Name: _____

Phone: _____

Notes:

_____

_____

_____

_____

Name: _____

Phone: _____

Notes:

_____

_____

_____

_____

Name: _____

Phone: _____

Notes:

_____

_____

_____

_____

Name: _____

Phone: _____

Notes:

_____

_____

_____

_____

Name: _____

Phone: _____

Notes:

_____

_____

_____

_____

Felicia Martin

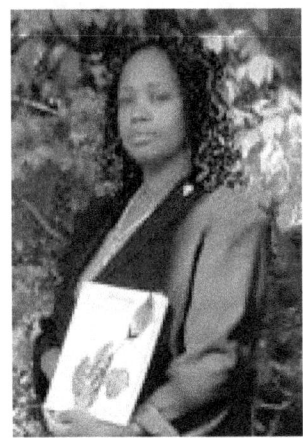

Her books:

Floetry "flowing like poetry"
Published April 2008

Reviewed as:
- A literary soundtrack for your day off
- A peaceful read
- It's like sitting on the porch with an old friend, reminiscing

Available on Amazon.com
Target.com
And many others

Love Jones
To be released in the Fall of 2008

Her websites:

Floetry.vpweb.com
Goodreads.com
Myspace.com/one_floetry_place
Beadedtreasures.50megs.com